Table of Contents

Introduction 2

History And Culture 2

   Methods Of Psilocybin Use.. 5

   Street Names For Psilocybin.. 6

The Story Of Magic Mushrooms 7

   Types Of Psychedelic Mushrooms.................................. 8

   Psilocybin Side Effects 9

What Are Psilocybin Mushrooms.................................. 10

   Other Mushrooms That Can Be Used As Natural Treatments
.... 12

   Physical Effects 14

   Enhancement And Suppression Cycles.......................... 19

   Amazing Health Benefits Of Psilocybin Mushrooms 21

   Long-Term Medical And Spiritual Benefits.......................... 24

   Disadvantages Of Magic Mushrooms............................... 26

   How To Grow Magic Mushrooms................................... 27

   Requirements For Growing Magic Mushrooms 28

   Easy Steps To Grow Magic Mushrooms 29

Psilocybin (4-phosphoryloxy-N,N-dimethyltryptamine) and psilocin are chemical compounds obtained from certain types of dried or fresh hallucinogenic mushrooms found in Mexico, South America and the southern and northwest regions of the United States. Psilocybin is classified as an indole-alkylamine (tryptamine). These compounds have similar structure to lysergic acid diethylamide (LSD), and are abused for their hallucinogenic and euphoric effects to produce a "trip".Hallucinogenic (psychedelic) effects are probably due to action on central nervous system serotonin (5-HT) receptors. There are over 180 species of mushrooms that contain the chemicals psilocybin or psilocin. Like the peyote (mescaline), hallucinogenic mushrooms have been used in native or religious rites for centuries.Both psilocybin and psilocin can also be produced synthetically in the lab.There have been reports that psilocybin bought on the streets can actually be other species of mushrooms laced with LSD.

History And Culture

There is evidence that suggests that psilocybin mushrooms have been used by humans in religious ceremonies for thousands of years. Murals dated 9000 to 7000 BCE found in the Sahara desert in southeast Algeria depict horned beings dressed as dancers holding mushroom-like objects. 6,000-year-old pictographs discovered near the Spanish town of Villar del Humo illustrate several mushrooms that have been tentatively identified as Psilocybe hispanica, a hallucinogenic species native to the area. Archaeological artifacts from Mexico have also been interpreted by some scholars as evidence for ritual and ceremonial usage of psychoactive mushrooms in the Mayan and Aztec cultures of Mesoamerica.[citation needed] In Nahuatl, the language of the Aztecs, the mushrooms were called teonanácatl,or "God's flesh". Following the arrival of Spanish explorers to the New World in the 16th century, chroniclers reported the use of mushrooms by the natives for ceremonial and religious purposes. Accounts describe mushrooms being eaten in festivities for the accession of emperors and the celebration of successful business trips by merchants. After the defeat of the Aztecs, the Spanish forbade traditional religious practices and rituals that they considered "pagan idolatry", including ceremonial mushroom use. For the next four centuries, the Indians of Mesoamerica hid their use of entheogens from the Spanish authorities.[citation needed] American banker and amateur ethnomycologist R. Gordon Wasson studied the ritual use of psychoactive mushrooms by the native population of a Mazatec village in Mexico. In 1957, Wasson described the psychedelic visions that he experienced during these rituals in "Seeking the Magic Mushroom", an article published in the popular American weekly Life magazine. Later the same year they were accompanied on a follow-up expedition by French mycologist Roger Heim, who identified several of the mushrooms as Psilocybe species. Heim cultivated the mushrooms in France, and sent samples for analysis to Albert Hofmann, a chemist employed by the Swiss pharmaceutical company Sandoz (now Novartis). Hofmann, who had in 1938 created LSD, led a research group that isolated and identified the psychoactive compounds from Psilocybe mexicana. He and his colleagues later synthesized a number of compounds chemically related to the naturally occurring psilocybin, to see how structural changes would affect psychoactivity. These included 4-HO-DET and 4-AcO-DMT.Sandoz marketed and sold pure psilocybin under the name Indocybin to physicians and clinicians worldwide without any reports of serious complications. In the early 1960s, Harvard University became a testing ground for psilocybin, through the efforts of Timothy Leary and his associates Ralph Metzner and Richard Alpert.Leary obtained synthesized psilocybin from Hofmann through Sandoz pharmaceutical. Some studies, such as the Concord Prison Experiment, suggested promising results using psilocybin in clinical psychiatry.Leary and Alpert's zealous advocacy for widespread hallucinogen use led to a well-publicized termination from Harvard. In response to concerns about the increase in unauthorized use of psychedelic substances by the general public, psilocybin and other hallucinogens received negative press and faced increasingly restrictive laws. In the United States, laws were passed in 1966 that prohibited the production, trade, or ingestion of hallucinogenic substances. Sandoz stopped producing LSD and psilocybin the same year.Further backlash against LSD usage swept psilocybin along with it into the Schedule I category of illicit substances in 1970. Subsequent restrictions on the use of these substances in human research made funding for such projects difficult to obtain, and scientists who worked with psychedelic drugs faced being "professionally marginalized".

Methods Of Psilocybin Use

- "Magic Mushrooms" have long, slender stems which may appear white or greyish topped by caps with dark gills on the underside. Dried mushrooms are usually a reddish rust brown color with isolated areas of off-white. Mushrooms are ingested orally and may be made into a tea or mixed into other foods. The mushrooms may be used as fresh or dried product. Psilocybin has a bitter, unpalatable taste.

- A "bad trip", or a unpleasant or even terrifying experience, may occur with any dose of psilocybin. In general, dried mushrooms contain about 0.2% to 0.4% psilocybin and only trace amounts of psilocin. The typical dose of psilocybin used for recreational purposes varies, with peak effects occurring in 1 to 2 hours, and lasting for about six hours.

- Dose and effects can vary considerably depending upon mushroom type, method of preparation, and tolerance of the individual. It can be difficult to determine the exact species of mushroom or how much hallucinogen each mushroom contains. Initial smaller doses and a longer period of time to determine the effects may be a safer option if you choose to use psilocybin for recreational purposes.

Street Names For Psilocybin

Drug dealers rarely sell psilocybin under its real name. Instead, the drug may be sold as:

- Magic mushrooms

- Shrooms

- Boomers

- Zoomers

- Mushies

- Simple simon

- Little smoke

- Sacred mushrooms

- Purple passion

- Mushroom soup

- Cubes

The Story Of Magic Mushrooms

Beginnings

The first use of hallucinogenic mushrooms dates back about 3,000 years to Mexico.They are still used by native people in some areas for religious ceremonies and healing, although the local communities encountered many struggles in the past. Shortly after the European conquest of these territories, magic mushrooms were banned for the first time in the early 17th century A couple of centuries passed before these mushrooms gained the attention of Western scientists and doctors for the first time. Robert Wasson, an American ethnomycologist, popularized these mushrooms in the 50s after returning from an expedition to Mexico where he participated in an indigenous Mazatec religious ritual. He was one of the first Westerners to participate in such a ritual. He published an article in the Life magazine called "Seeking The Magic Mushroom" in which he described his experience.The book became extremely popular, especially in the counterculture movement of the time, and led many people to travel Mexico seeking to experience the same.But this only brought devastation and unwanted attention from foreigners and police to the local community.Luckily, it also brought some attention from the scientific community. Psilocybin was first isolated, identified, and synthesized by Albert Hofmann, the "father of LSD", in the late 50s (from P. mexicana).He later summarized his thoughts about psychedelics, including LSD and psilocybin, in the book "LSD – My Problem Child"

Types Of Psychedelic Mushrooms

There are over 100 species of psychedelic mushrooms, but the best-known ones are

- Psilocybe azurescens (highest psilocybin content)
- Psilocybe bohemica (second highest psilocybin content)
- Conocbe cyanopus

- Copelandia cyanescens

- Panaeolus africanus

- Panaeolus subbalteus

- Inocybe aeruginascens

- Psilocybe cubensis

- Psilocybe cyanescens

- Psilocybe mexicana

- Psilocybe semilanceata

- Psilocybe tampanensis

- Psilocybin vs LSD or Mescaline

Psilocybin Side Effects

Clinical Trials

- Given in a supportive, controlled, psychotherapeutic environment, psilocybin does not cause any serious adverse effects. Higher doses of psilocybin are more likely to cause anxiety or fear due to feelings of ego dissolution or lack of control. In one trial of 18 people, higher doses caused the following:

- 39% experienced extreme fear, fear of insanity or felt trapped

- 44% reported delusions or paranoid thinking

- Ultimately, nobody reported a decrease of wellbeing or life satisfaction from the overall experience.

Other Adverse Effects That Occurred In Clinical Studies Include:

- Dizziness
- A slight increase in blood pressure or heart rate
- Unusual body sensations
- Mood changes
- Fatigue and yawning

What Are Psilocybin Mushrooms

Psilocybin mushrooms are actually known as Psilocybe cubensis.They're the scientific name for more than 100 mushroom species that contain psilocybin and psilocin. These two compounds account for the hallucinations and "tripping" that occur when a person ingests these mushrooms.While psychedelic mushrooms and hallucinogens seem like a relic from a hippie, Grateful Dead-loving past, they're giving doctors new hope in treating a range of mental health issues. Like so most drugs and chemicals that alter the mind, researchers aren't yet exactly sure psilocybin works. What they do know, however, is that when psilocybin reaches the brain, it decreases brain activity, particularly in the medial prefrontal cortex (mPFC) and the posterior cingulate cortex (PCC).The mPFC is associated with obsessive thinking and, in people with depression, is usually overactive. In fact, antidepressants all stifle mPFC. The PCC, on the other hand, is believed to play a role in consciousness, ego and sense of self. Psilocybin seems to quiet down the "noise" in a person's brain, letting them access parts of their mind that are normally stifled.It also seems to affect serotonin, the neurotransmitter linked to moods, anxiety and depression. One researcher likened psilocybin to "inverse PTSD."But instead of a traumatizing incident haunting patients, instead, the psilocybin mushrooms create a really positive memory they can turn to for months. In fact, during the 1950s and '60s, hallucinogens like psilocybin were being studied for their potential in the psychiatry and oncology fields.However, in 1970, the Controlled Substances Act was signed into law. It categorized hallucinogens like psilocybin mushrooms as a Schedule 1 drug, meaning it has a high potential for abuse and has no currently accepted medical use in treatment in the U.S. Federal funds for research dried up. Most studies being done now are largely funded by non-profits and private donors who believe in the drug's potential. And these latest studies show there is a lot of potential to be explored.

Other Mushrooms That Can Be Used As Natural Treatments

But there are ways to use mushrooms as natural treatments legally, of course.Your favorite mushroom: With more than 200 mushroom species available, you're bound to have a favorite. Luckily, mushrooms in general are fantastic for you. They're low in carbs, calories and fat, but packed with antioxidants and B vitamins.They're known to increase immunity and lower inflammation, the root of most diseases. They're also known to lower LDL, "bad" cholesterol, while increasing HDL, the good kind.And since most of us aren't getting enough natural sunlight, they're also great in preventing vitamin D deficiencies.

Cordyceps: While not technically mushrooms, cordyceps are renowned for their ability to fight free radicals and are great disease-fighting mushrooms.In fact, some studies have shown that cordyceps sometimes can behave like natural cancer treatments, preventing tumor growth.

Maitake

Maitake mushrooms are known for stimulating the immune system, thanks to specialized components found in them.In fact, in Asia, they're often used in conjunction with other types of cancer treatment, and can even help minimize the effects of chemotherapy or radiation. They've also been linked to balancing hormones naturally. It improves stamina and acts like a natural aphrodisiac, too.

Oyster

Oyster mushrooms are an anti-inflammatory food and are exceptionally good at reducing joint pain. They strengthen blood vessel walls and can help increase iron levels, especially helpful if you don't eat too much meat.

Reishi

Reishi mushrooms have been a superfood for thousands of years.They have adaptogen herb-like properties to deal with the negative properties of stress.But best of all, reishi mushrooms are known to protect against inflammation, autoimmune disorders and heart disease.They also increase the release of the body's natural killer cells.

Shiitake

Not only are shiitake mushrooms delicious, but they're awesome at protecting our DNA from oxidative damage. Excitingly for plant-lovers, shiitake mushrooms also contain all of the eight essential amino acids our bodies need but don't produce on their own.They're known for boosting the immune system and might even fight cancer cells.

Turkey Tail

These colorful mushrooms are one of the most common, and that's a good thing. They're known to treat the common cold and flu. It's also being trialed as a way to build up the immune system for cancer patients going through chemotherapy.

Physical Effects

Sedation

Psilocybin is reported to be relaxing, stoning and mildly sedating. This sense of sedation is often accompanied by compulsive yawning.

Spontaneous Bodily Sensations

The "body high" of psilocybin can be described as a pleasurable, soft and all-encompassing tingling sensation or glow. This maintains a consistent presence that steadily rises with the onset and hits its limit once the peak has been reached. Once the peak of the experience or sensation is reached it can feel incredibly euphoric and tranquil or heavy and immobilizing depending on the dose.

Perception Of Bodily Heaviness

This effect corresponds to the general sense of sedation and relaxation that characterizes psilocybin experiences, this manifests as a bodily heaviness that discourages movement but is typically only prominent during the first half of the experience. This particular physical effect seems to be more commonly experienced and pronounced with certain "woodlover" species of mushrooms such as Psilocybe azurescens.

Tactile Enhancement

This effect is less prominent than with that of LSD or 2C-B but is still present and unique in its character. It is repeatedly described as feeling very primitive in its nature often times with the small hairs on the user's arms or legs feeling slightly itchy or even ticklish against the skin.

Changes In Felt Bodily Form

This effect is often accompanied by a sense of warmth or unity and usually occurs around the peak of the experience or directly after.Users can feel as if they are physically part of or conjoined with other objects.This is usually reported as feeling comfortable in its sensations and even peaceful.

Nausea

This effect can be greatly lessened or even completely avoided if the individual has an empty stomach prior to ingestion. It is often recommended that one either refrain from eating for approximately 6 to 8 hours beforehand, or eat a light meal 3 to 4 hours before if they are feeling physically fatigued.

Excessive Yawning

This effect seems to be uniquely pronounced among psilocybin and related tryptamines. It can occur to a lesser degree on LSD and very rarely on psychedelic phenethylamines like mescaline.It typically occurs in combination with watery eyes.

- Watery eyes
- Frequent urination
- Muscle contractions
- Olfactory hallucination
- Pupil dilation

- Runny nose

- Increased salivation

Brain Zaps

Although this effect is very rare, it can still occur for those susceptible to it.This component is however much less common and intense than it is with serotonin releasing agents such as MDMA.

Seizure

This is a rare effect but can happen in a small population of those who are predisposed to them, particularly while in physically taxing conditions such as being dehydrated, undernourished, overheated, or fatigued.

Cognitive Effects

The cognitive effects and general head space of psilocybin is described by many as extremely relaxing, profound and stoning in style when compared to other commonly used psychedelics such as LSD or 2C-B which tend to be energetic and stimulating, it is also regarded as being significantly less clearheaded than other commonly used tryptamines such as DMT and ayahuasca.

Emotion Enhancement

This effect can be described as being more prominent, consistent and profound when compared to other traditional psychedelics such as mescaline or LSD.This can lead to strong feelings of compassion, urgency and even completely sporadic moments of intense emotional significance that can also be periodically affected by enhancement and suppression cycles.

Empathy, Affection, And Sociability Enhancement

This effect differs from MDMA and other entactogens in that it isn't as central to the experience, feels less forced and more natural and is experienced at a less consistent rate. The sociability enhancement in particular only occurs rarely and it appears to be more emotional.

Language Suppression

This effect can be described as a perceived inability or general unwillingness to talk aloud despite feeling perfectly capable of formulating coherent thoughts within one's internal narrative.It is much more common among inexperienced users.

Analysis Enhancement

This effect is consistent in its manifestation and outrospection dominant.

Enhancement And Suppression Cycles

This can be described as constant waves of extremely stimulated and profound thinking which are spontaneously surpassed in a cyclic fashion by waves of general thought suppression and mental intoxication. These two states seem to switch between each other in a consistent loop once every 20 to 60 minutes.

Feelings of impending doom. This effect is usually only experienced during the come up phase but typically completely passes or subsides once the primary effects begin. It should be noted that this effect is relatively consistent and normal for psilocybin and related tryptamines which is why a positive and well-informed mindset is key. Less regularly this aspect can also occur during the peak but will most often be met afterwards with sensations of euphoria, catharsis or rejuvenation.

Cognitive Euphoria

- Autonomous voice communication
- Suggestibility enhancement
- Conceptual thinking
- Thought connectivity
- Thought deceleration

- Thought loops

- Thought organization

Other Effects Of Hallucinogenic Drugs Can Include:

- Intensified Feelings And Sensory Experiences

- Changes In Sense Of Time (For Example, Time Passing By Slowly)

- Increased Blood Pressure, Breathing Rate, Or Body Temperature

- Loss Of Appetite

- Dry Mouth

- Sleep Problems

- Mixed Senses (Such As "Seeing" Sounds Or "Hearing" Colors)

- Spiritual Experiences

- Feelings Of Relaxation Or Detachment From Self/Environment

- Uncoordinated Movements

- Lowered Inhibition

- Excessive Sweating

- Panic

- Paranoia - Extreme And Unreasonable Distrust Of Others

- Psychosis - Disordered Thinking Detached From Reality

Amazing Health Benefits Of Psilocybin Mushrooms

Psilocybin mushrooms might just be the "next best thing" in holistic healing and wellness.

High CBC Full Spectrum Gut, Microbiome, and Brain Function Formula.Also known as "magic mushrooms", there are more than 200 types of mushrooms with psychoactive properties. These mushrooms have been used ceremonially for thousands of years in various parts of the world but only recently the Western world has encountered its tremendous healing effects, both medical as well as psychological and emotional. There are more and more studies out there which are proving that psilocybin mushrooms are far from what the government considers them to be a "Schedule 1" drug, addictive and harmful. Here are some of the most important health benefits psilocybin mushrooms can offer you.

Facts on Psilocybin Mushrooms

- **Stimulates Growth Of New Brain Cells**

Particles Asymmetrical Branching Fractal network, Nerves, neurons , blood vessels, capillaries growing 3d render. A study conducted by the University of South Florida published in 2013 studied the effects of psilocybin mushrooms on fear-conditioned mice.

- **What They Discovered Startled Them**

The main ingredient in psilocybin mushrooms, psilocybin, empowered the mice to get over their fear and promoted new neurons growth and regeneration in their brains. Memory, learning, and the ability to relearn that a once threatening stimuli is no longer a danger absolutely depends on the ability of the brain to alter its connections.We believe that neuroplasticity plays a critical role in psilocybin accelerating fear extinction.It is highly possible that in the future we will continue these studies since many interesting questions have come up from these experiments. The hope is that we can extend the findings to humans in clinical trials.

- **Reduces Pain Due To Social Rejection**

We all go through rejection from time to time, right?It is a natural process when it comes to interacting with other individuals. A study performed by a team of Swiss neurobiologists, published in April 2016, stated that psilocybin is of great help in reducing the pain resulting from social rejection.

- **Alleviates OCD Symptoms**

Obsessive-compulsive disorder (also known as OCD) is a psychiatric disorder which is occurring especially in patients suffering from schizophrenia, bipolar disorders and other psychiatric ailments. A study performed by the University of Arizona in 2006 discovered that psilocybin mushrooms are very effective in alleviating the symptoms of this disorder.

- **Soothes Anxiety**

In a 2011 study, researcher's discovered that advanced-stage patient's suffering from cancer would have their anxiety soothed and drastically lowered after being administered psilocybin mushrooms.

- **Lowers Depression**

Studies have shown that psilocybin mushrooms are effective at treating depression very effectively, as well as treating post-traumatic stress disorder. Psilocybin, the active ingredient in psychoactive mushrooms, has provided the spiritual and cultural bedrock of many great civilisations. The Aztecs referred to teonanácatl, which translates as 'divine mushroom', and modern neuroscience has revealed how psilocybin interacts with serotonin receptors in the brain in order to produce a range of consciousness-altering effects.

Long-Term Medical And Spiritual Benefits

There was a famous study done at Johns Hopkins University which left researchers stunned.Out of 36 test subjects, a third said that their experience was the most significant (spiritual) experience of their lives, while over two thirds stated that it was definitely in their top five most significant life experiences.

Psilocybin is an amazing tool for unlocking the mysteries of human consciousness. The core feature of this mystical experience is a strong sense of inter-connectedness to all things, a rising sense of self-confidence, clarity and communal responsibility, altruism and social justice. Understanding the nature of these effects and their consequences, may very well be the key to survival of the human species.

Connecting The Brain In New Ways

Functional MRIs performed during the psychedelic experience induced by psilocybin mushrooms suggest that these "magic mushrooms" wire different parts of the brain together, facilitating a much smoother communication between its various parts.

Smoking Cessation And Other Addictions

If you are caught up with unhealthy patterns in your life psychedelics can help. Magic mushrooms have been shown to help treat addiction to habit-forming drugs like cocaine and nicotine.In 2008, Amanda Feilding of The Beckley Foundation initiated a collaboration with Johns Hopkins University on a pilot study investigating psilocybin-assisted psychotherapy to overcome nicotine addiction.With continued support from the Heffter Research Institute, the ongoing research is strengthening the case for psilocybin as a breakthrough treatment for substance abuse disorders.

Psychological Distress Caused By Cancer

Preliminary results are due on studies involving psilocybin's effects on treating anxiety in people that have advanced-stage cancer. A trial at Johns Hopkins in 2016 was responsible for finding that even a single dose of psilocybin greatly decreased depression in people that were diagnosed with cancer that was life threatening.

Cessation Of Addiction To Smoking And Cessation To Other Addictions

While the study was small, researchers at a Johns Hopkins University Trusted Source found that therapies of psilocybin helped in abstaining from smoking.

Psilocybin is also said to treat alternative addictions, including an addiction to cocaine and to alcohol.

Disadvantages Of Magic Mushrooms

Mental Illness

When magic mushrooms are consumed by people that suffer from a variety of mental illnesses – schizophrenia or panic disorder, for example – it can bring about behavior patterns that are highly erratic and dangerous.

Nausea

When magic mushrooms are consumed, even in smaller quantities, they can cause nausea and upset stomach. It can also cause vomiting though only when the mushrooms are in a decayed state. When vomiting occurs, it's not caused by psylocibin. Rather, it is because of bacteria or contaminated microbes.

Fear

Feelings of fear, uneasiness and paranoia have been reported from magic mushroom "users."Further, "shrooms" can bring about visual imagery and auditory hallucinations. Shroom users may well be entirely aware of what they are hearing and what they are seeing, but magic mushrooms can cause doubt as to authenticity and reality.

Physical Weakness

Shrooms can cause a feeling of being physically weak and even immobile.

How To Grow Magic Mushrooms

For Propagation Through Spores

Cut the stems of magic mushroom and place it on a clean piece of wax paper, keeping the caps gill-side-down. Cover the caps with a cup and let it rest for 24 hours. Next, take a wide clean plastic container and fill it with a nutrient-rich soil (you can make it yourself by mixing equal parts of peat moss, sterile compost, and potting soil).Transfer the spores carefully to the container and cover the top with a transparent cellophane layer. Make 8-10 holes in plastic wrap to allow enough airflow in the growing pot and mist the soil with water, as they flourish in humidity.

Requirements For Growing Magic Mushrooms

Location

Mushrooms don't need as much sunlight, like other plants, for growth and food. Thus, the best place to grow them is a basement or any dark area, as darkness retains moisture that their spores use for reproduction.

Moisture

Just like all fungi, mushrooms also flourish in moist climates. Hence they need damp and humid growing media, such as compost or manure. Also, mist the soil to maintain moisture.

Temperature

The ideal temperature for growing magic mushrooms is 65-75F (18-24C). Keep them away from the cool breeze and dry air, as it can kill or restrict them from growing.

Nourishment

Mushrooms need starch, sugar, fats, nitrogen, protein, and lignin to grow well. To fulfill their need for these nutrients, you can use compost made from straw and manure. If you don't have these materials, you can use corn, peat moss, and sand.They are also capable of extracting essential nutrients from the wood of logs or sawdust.

Easy Steps To Grow Magic Mushrooms

Lighting

One of the most important factors when growing magic mushrooms is the amount of light that they receive and the quality of that light – they should never be given direct light. They can be grown using sunlight or a normal white bulb, but never directly on the substrate. In as far as the amount of light needed.This can be tricky, as mushrooms naturally grow on the ground in large forests, spending lots of time in the dark. If you grow them using sunlight, all you have to do is leave your curtains open and place the mushrooms to one side of the window, making sure that they're never in direct sunlight. If you're using a light in your house you'll need to position it so that the light doesn't directly shine on the substrate.

Humidity

Humidity is essential, as it's what activates the mycelium which is where the shrooms sprout from. In order to provide the right amount of humidity, you'll need to use a small greenhouse propagator. Hydrate the substrate using bottled or osmosis water – never use tap water. When you add water, the substrate will begin swelling up, so you'll need to go slowly to make sure that it's evenly wet. Once it's been fully soaked, remove any leftover water – if there's any water left at the bottom of the container it may cause fungi. Our mushroom kits come with a bag that you can use as a propagator, although if you want the best possible results we recommend getting a proper greenhouse propagator. In order to activate the mycelium you'll need to keep humidity at a steady 90% for at least two days inside the propagator.This means that you'll need to add some extra water to the bottom of your propagator not the container with the substrate. Make sure this water is also osmosis or bottled.Another way to do this is by keeping the lid on the containers, which concentrates humidity a lot more. After the first two days you'll need to lower humidity to around 70%, which is easy to do by fiddling with the little windows on the side of your propagator.

Temperature

Temperature is another incredibly important parameter; mushrooms generally thrive between 21 and 24°C, so if you want to produce as many shrooms as possible we recommend keeping the propagator right in the middle. If it's cold where you're planning on growing them, you can always get a heated propagator or a heated blanket for underneath your propagator. If you grow your mushrooms under 21°C they'll grow much slower and produce less shrooms – once the mycelium is active, it only has a certain amount of time to produce mushrooms.

Hygiene

Last but not least, hygiene and a clean environment is paramount to growing magic mushrooms. They're quite sensitive, and they need a clean and sterilized environment – never ever touch them with your hands, make sure to use latex gloves when handling the kit at all time and, if possible, a facemask. You need to try and avoid altering the atmosphere around them as much as possible – don't smoke, use deodorant or any other kind of spray product in the room that they're in or they may become contaminated and not grow properly. Give your magic mushroom kits the right lighting, humidity, temperature and clean environment and they'll produce plenty of psychedelic heads.

And also gather the following equipment and ingredients:

- 12 Wide mouth half-pint jars with lids (make sure to get wide mouth)
- Cup for measuring
- Hammer and small nail
- Large mixing bowl and spoon
- Strainer
- Tin foil (heavy duty)
- Large cooking pot with a tight lid (or an Instant Pot)
- Small towel
- Microspore tape
- Clear plastic storage box 50 – 115 L
- ¼ inch drill bit/Drill
- Perlite
- Mist spray bottle

Ingredients

- Spore syringe, 10-12 cc (you might use this brand)
- Organic brown rice or brown rice flour (use a coffee grinder for brown rice)
- Vermiculite, medium/fine
- Drinking water (preferably distilled)

Sanitation Items

- 70% Isopropyl alcohol and lysol (or similar)

- Bic lighter (or propane torch)

- Air sanitizer

- Latex gloves, surgical mask, and glove box (optional)

www.ingramcontent.com/pod-product-compliance
Lightning Source LLC
Chambersburg PA
CBHW051408150726
48000CB00003B/1386